KETO DIET COOKBOOK 2019:

THE PERFECT AND COMPLETE KETO COOKBOOK WITH HIGH FAT/LOW CARB DIET PLANS.

BY PHILIP KOCH.

TABLE OF CONTENTS.

WHY YOU SHOULD READ THIS BOOK.

You are struggling with the idea of coming up with a keto meal prep.

You are probably tired of making hard decisions when it comes to choosing what to eat for breakfast, lunch or dinner.

You have a burning desire to get into keto diet and plan to make it successful.

Now you want a simple way out with complete and detailed guidelines on how to go about the keto diet meal prep. Well here is a collection of details governing meal prepping.

This book contains the details you want.

INTRODUCTION.

The most fulfilling way to actually find success in ketogenic diet is by having a meal plan for the whole week or month depending on how long you want it.

The best meal plan is to have a weekly one since you'll have to be held responsible for the daily follow up.

Meal prep is essential when it comes to fitness and nutrition if you want to set yourself up for success. Planning and laying down the foot notes for your meals in advance can save you the negative behaviors, such as grabbing some sugary and high carb foods, which are contrary to what you want to achieve.

Having meal prep can actually have some benefits to you. It can save you time when going through the recipe and deciding what to buy. This will also increase the chances upon which you will stick to the diet.

Research has been conducted regarding the incorporation of the use of meal prep and it has been concluded that planning has a significant increase in the likelihood of achieving success compare to just being motivated to engage into a healthy diet.

In case you need some solid/convincing reasons as to why having a meal plan is such important if you want to lose weight, we got you covered.

Reasons for having a meal plan.

Saves time and money.

Committing a couple of hours weekly towards meal preparation can be a savior when it comes to shopping, picking meals and cooking. It can also save you on the waste of food.

To ensure that you stick to the essentials and use everything you planned to use, meal plan is the golden tool.

Helps achieve ketosis.

The only difficulty that can be experienced in ketogenic diets is the calculation of macros, but by incorporating a keto friendly meal plan, there is a chance of sticking to the macro goals.

Helps in decision making.

Indecision or decision fatigue is normal behavior exhibited by human beings. This often happens mainly because there are more decisions that need to be made on a daily basis and there is a less likelihood to make the right ones. Therefore, making time to come up with a meal plan can save your brain juice during the week and you will be able to focus on other decisions.

Having successful meal prep requires some of the important ingredients and basic equipment. It is good to invest in quality equipment that give you flexibility and accuracy in the kitchen.

Here are some of the equipments to invest in.

Skillet.

Chef's knife.

Blender.

Crockpot.

Vegetable spiralizer.

Immersion blender.

Kitchen scale.

By preparing your meals ahead of time, you are no longer preparing to fail but rather preparing to excel in your health and weight loss journey.

Bottom line, meal prepping takes the guesswork out of what you're going to eat for each meal.

The time you normally spend in the kitchen every day and is now spent on the other things you've always been ignoring in life.

Steps for easy keto meal prep.

Truth be told, no one likes rules but its important to have some rules or guidelines if at all you want to achieve anything. The following structure explains a simple strategy to follow when getting into meal prep.

Decide what to eat.

You have to make a date to sit down and have an outline of whatever you are going to eat for the next one week based on the following points:

The kind of meals you will eat throughout the week for either breakfast, lunch of dinner. It is important to use recipes that the calories and macros are already listed, thus making it easy to be noticed.

Whether you will be having the same meal more than once.

The number of people eating the meal.

The recipe and the exact ingredients for every meal.

The days you will be shopping for the ingredients and to actually cook the meals.

Make a shopping list.

Have a compilation of your shopping list basing in the ingredients named from each recipe. Break the list down into categories excluding the exact amounts of each ingredient but by actually shopping for the whole foods.

Cook the meals.

Like everything else, cooking gets ugly at first but it can only get better with time. The key is to always practice. Make sure to have read the whole recipe and ensure that all the ingredients in place before starting.

Upon cooking all the meals you can now go ahead and separate them into different containers to go daily for the whole week.

Planning and prepping meals early will definitely make everything easier in any day as it saves your time, money and the hassle all week. It also help you stick to the diet and find the rhythm that will work for you successfully.

HOW TO ACTUALLY CREATE A KETO MEAL PREP.

When it comes to actually creating a working keto meal prep plan, the first step can sometimes be hard to take. Here is a clear layout of what you might want to do:

Set a goal.

You have to know the ultimate goal for getting into this diet. Whether it is to lose weight, health improvement, and mental clarity or to boost your immune system.

This has to be written down as it is a way of making a commitment to pursue the results.

Calculation of macros.

The ratio of macronutrients is a vital thing to do in keto diet. A macro calculator can be used in figuring out the content of fat, protein and carbs needed

You have to always remember the following range of the macros to be used,

Low carb 5-10%

Protein 20-25%

High fat 70-80%

By putting the above ranges in mind, you will have easy time determining how much can be taken in each category depending on your lifestyle and body configuration.

Planning the meals.

Your plan for meals is dependent on the daily macros either for each day or the whole week.

You should be able to plan well if you will be eating keto for breakfast, lunch or dinner. Once you have planned the meals, a shopping list with ingredients needed for each meal.

Shopping.

Focus on the healthiest foods resist any junkies and above all, stick to the list.

Go for it.

Now your ingredients are on check and you have the meal planned, the next thing is to go for what works best for you. What meets your specifications?

You can cook and store for the whole week or better still can be cooked daily for each meal.

For example,

Day 1:

Breakfast. Serving chocolate pancakes with blueberry butter.

Macros;

Fat 57g

Carbs 12g

Protein 27g

Calories 611.

Lunch; Chicken salad (crispy cheesy)

Macros;

Fat 36g

Carbs 8g

Protein55g

Calories 575

Dinner; Grilled ribeye steak.

Macros;

Fat 62g

Carbs 1g

Protein 20g

Calories 636

Macros for the day;

Fat 155g

Carbs 21g

Protein 102g

Calories 1822

KETOGENIC DIET FOODS.

The following are some of the ketogenic foods split into the respective categories.

FATS.

 Whether saturated or mono unsaturated.

Avocado

Egg yolks

Coconut oil, Olive oil or Avocado oil.

Nuts and seeds.

Coconut butter.

Macadamia nuts.

Ghee.

Fatty fish.

For the poly-unsaturated fats, you need an effective balance between omega 3s and omega 6s. These are essential fatty acids that must be acquired from the diet.

The omega elements are important in ensuring proper nerve and brain functionality. They also reduce risks associated with heart disease, type 2 diabetes and the decline in brain function at old age.

Too much of omega 6 can cause some side effects like body inflammations mainly due to excess use of peanuts and plant oils.

VEGETABLES.

When choosing vegetables you will have to consider the non-starchy, low carb and should have to be leafy greens.

Lettuce.

Broccoli

Spinach.

Kale.

Brussels sprouts.

Cauliflower.

Zucchini.

Spaghetti squash.

Onions.

Bell peppers.

Asparagus.

Cucumber.

FRUITS.

When choosing the fruits to be eaten, lower sugar options should be considered. They have to be taken in little amounts.

Taking fresh or organic fruits and vegetables if the best option.

These fruits are:

Blueberries.

Cherries.

Cranberries.

Raspberries.

Cranberries.

Malberries.

DAIRY PRODUCTS.

Organic or raw dairy products are most preferred since there is enough quantity of fat needed.

Pretty much all the dairy products are good for keto.

The following are some of the examples of the dairy products:

Heavy cream.

All forms of cheese.

Full fat yogurts.

Hard and soft cheese.

Sour cream.

Moyannaise

HERBS, SPICES AND SWEETENERS.

Most of the traditional seasoning contains a lot of sugars and carbs, thus, not keto friendly. So when getting seasonings, it is important to ensure that they are pure herbs or spices and doesn't contain any traces of sugars.

Examples of these ones are:

Parsley.

Oregano.

Basil.

Salt and pepper.

Cinnamon.

Nutmeg.

Chilli powder.

Lemon and lime juices.

When choosing sweeteners, you need to avoid sugary foods as much as you can but here are the tips to have in mind during the process of selection:

Low glycemic sweeteners are good since they won't contribute to the carb intake or interfere with the blood sugar level.

Sweeteners made from alcohol are not good for use in keto.

Here are some of the examples of sweeteners.

Liquid stevia.

Monk fruit.

Erythritol.

Xylitol.

SNACKS.

Ketogenic diet is often one of those diets that is very much easier to follow.

At times you might not need a snack at all, thus making it easier to limit it.

In an event that you genuinely feel hungry and you think that a snack will help with the macros, then you have every reason to have a few nuts or cheese but it is important to track the quantity of snacks you eat.

Make sure to always have small portions of the snack as possible.

The following are some examples of snacks you can use:

Eggs.

Cucumber.

Macadamia nuts.

Nonfat or full fat green yogurt.

Cherry tomatoes.

Almonds.

Cheese.

Olives.

DRINKS.

It's a little bit hard to know the kind of drinks to use on keto diet.

The best guess is to use water since it is the best take at any time.

Lemon water can be used to actually bring about neutrality of the blood pH since it alkalizes the acids.

Use of too much caffeine may bring about some side effects to the blood sugar levels, therefore, do not exceed 2 cups per day.

Alcohol is not recommended as it interferes with ketosis but wine can be taken if insisted or when attending occasions.

Below is the list of drinks on keto diet:

Black coffee.

Bone broth.

Almond milk.

Black or green tea.

Herbal tea.

FOODS TO AVOID ON KETO.

Soy products.

High carb fruits like; bananas, water melon, orange, papaya, grapes...

Fruit juices.

Legumes.

Gluten.

All sauces.

All starchy vegetables.

Grains.

Starchy foods.

Sugar and processed foods.

Hydrogenated oils.

Artificial sweeteners.

Sweetened beverages.

ADVANTAGES OF MEAL PREP.

Its time saving.

It takes less time to cook separate portions of the same meal at once as compared to cooking separate portions of the same meal each day.

It takes time cooking all the portions once but it will save you the hassle of cooking every day.

Its cheap.

Buying food and then cooking them in a bulk is good when it comes to saving money. This goes hand in hand with actually packing your food and avoid buying food in the cafeteria at work.

Helps in the daily decisions on what to eat.

Meal prep saves a lot of your 'brain juice' in decision making since most of the decisions made during the day involve what to eat. So the best thing to do is to concentrate all your energy for some 2 days to come up with a meal plan and save your energy for other things.

You can control the meal portions.

The measurements you make on each portion is good as it helps control the food served. You won't consume excess of what you are supposed to. With this you will avoid unnecessary food taken in between meals.

The main idea of controlling the portions is to actually have enough on a daily basis.

You can control your macros.

Planning what you will eat in advance will help track your macros without frequently measuring anything as time goes by.

You will be able to adjust wherever necessary as you have a good overview of the daily macros.

Makes it easy to have easily available delicious food.

This is due to the fact that you can adjust the taste and be able to control the quality and quantity of the ingredients used.

The end result is a delicious food that you need at your own comfort.

Enhances creative cooking.

Meal prepping doesn't have to be about having the same meal over and over again, its good though if you enjoy having the same thing consecutively.

Better still a few side dishes can be prepared to facilitate rotation or different salads can be eaten on different days of the week.

The key here is to be creative around all the ingredients and you will get some good foods.

TIPS FOR A SUCCESSFUL LOW CARB MEAL PREP.

Try new some new recipes once in a while.

You can at times try cooking two different things at once.

Always keep some frozen meals for emergency cases.

Try different methods of reheating or cooking meat; like adding a little fat.

When prepping snacks, make it simple as possible.

For salads, just have the ingredients ready but don't meal prep them to avoid withering.

Meal prep money saving hacks.

Let's be honest, the weekly shopping trips can be pretty much pricey.

Better still, there is a way that you can cook at home and save your money.

With these tips, you can actually keep your fridge full and save money at the same time.

1. Go for the produce in season.

Seasonal fruits and veggies are tastier and often cheaper.

2. Freeze any leftover smoothies into empty ice cream molds.
3. Buy the ingredients you want in bulk.
4. Compare prices to get best deals.
5. Go to the market in the evening.

When the vendors are ready to leave, they want to get rid of their produce so they won't hesitate to give you a good deal on food.

TAKE AWAY NOTES.

If you always run out of ideas about what to eat, you find yourself often busy and can't think of something to eat or you always struggle with staying under your calories, then you really have to give meal prep a try.

If you are busy during the week, you can actually meal prep the meals and snacks a few days at a time. Everything can just be done at once and save the rest of the days for other works.

Ketogenic diet involves completely natural healthy foods, therefore, you should not have the urge to take snacks or go above the calories required.

Make sure to eat all the foods prepared in order to make sure that you track the macros very well.

Keep everything simple and avoid processed foods as much as possible.